My Mediterranean Dash Diet Daily Recipes

A Set of Tasty and Affordable Recipes for Your Mediterranean Dash Diet Meals

Kathyrn Solano

© Copyright 2021 - All rights reserved.

The content contained within this book may not be reproduced, duplicated or transmitted without direct written permission from the author or the publisher.

Under no circumstances will any blame or legal responsibility be held against the publisher, or author, for any damages, reparation, or monetary loss due to the information contained within this book. Either directly or indirectly.

Legal Notice:

This book is copyright protected. This book is only for personal use. You cannot amend, distribute, sell, use, quote or paraphrase any part, or the content within this book, without the consent of the author or publisher.

Disclaimer Notice:

Please note the information contained within this document is for educational and entertainment purposes only. All effort has been executed to present accurate, up to date, and reliable, complete information. No warranties of any kind are declared or implied. Readers acknowledge that the author is not engaging in the rendering of legal, financial, medical or professional advice. The content within this book has been derived from various sources. Please consult a licensed professional before attempting any techniques outlined in this book.

By reading this document, the reader agrees that under no circumstances is the author responsible for any losses, direct or indirect, which are incurred as a result of the use of information contained within this document, including, but not limited to, — errors, omissions, or inaccuracies.

Table of contents

LUNCH AND DINNER RECIPES 6

    Carrot Soup With Parmesan Croutons 6
    Greek Baked Cod 9
    Pistachio Sole Fish 11
    Beef Tomato Soup 13
    Baked Tilapia 15
    Herbal Lamb Cutlets With Roasted Veggies 17
    A Great Mediterranean Snapper 19
    Mediterranean Snapper 21
    Italian Skillet Chicken With Mushrooms And Tomatoes 23
    Red Wine–braised Pot Roast With Carrots And Mushrooms 26
    Zoodles With Turkey Meatballs 28
    Italian Platter 30
    Mediterranean Pizza 32
    Roasted Vegetable Quinoa Bowl 34
    Mediterranean Salmon 38
    Heartthrob Mediterranean Tilapia 40
    Garlic And Cajun Shrimp Bowl With Noodles 42
    Garlic Marinated Chicken 44
    Tabouli Salad 46
    Mediterranean Flounder 48
    Greek Lemon Chicken Soup 50
    Mediterranean Steamed Salmon With Fresh Herbs And Lemon 52
    Grilled Salmon Tzatziki Bowl 55
    Smoky Chickpea, Chard, And Butternut Squash Soup 58
    Herbed Tuna Salad Wraps 60
    Mediterranean Potato Salad 62
    Mediterranean Zucchini Noodles 64
    Lobster Salad 66

GREAT MEDITERRANEAN DIET RECIPES 67

    Red lentil soup 67
    Salmon soup 69
    Falafel sandwiches 71
    Roasted tomato basil soup 72
    Greek black-eyed peas stew 74
    Juicy salmon burgers 76
    Braised eggplant and chickpeas 78

- Mediterranean tuna salad sandwiches 80
- Moroccan vegetable tagine 82
- Mediterranean grilled balsamic chicken with olive tapenade 84
- Linguine and zucchini noodles with shrimp 86
- Chicken gyros with Tzatziki sauce 88
- Greek chicken marinade 90
- Mediterranean chicken quinoa bowl with broccoli and tomato 91
- Chicken piccata 93
- Chopped grilled vegetable with farro 95
- 30 minutes' pork scaloppini with lemons and capers 97
- Greek chicken kebabs 99
- Shrimp pasta with roasted red peppers and artichokes 101
- 30 minutes Caprese chicken 103
- Greek turkey burgers with Tzatziki sauce 105
- Saucy Greek baked shrimp 107

LUNCH AND DINNER RECIPES

Carrot Soup With Parmesan Croutons

Servings: 4

Cooking Time: 25 To 30 Minutes

Ingredients:

2 cups vegetable broth, no salt added, and low sodium is best

1 teaspoon dried thyme

¼ teaspoon sea salt

1 ounce grated parmesan cheese

2 pounds of carrots, unpeeled

2 tablespoons extra virgin olive oil

½ chopped onion

2 ½ cups water

¼ teaspoon crushed red pepper

4 slices of whole-grain bread

Directions:

Cut your carrots into ½-inch slices

Take one rack from your oven and place it four inches from the broiler heating element. One either rack, place two large-rimmed baking sheets and turn your oven to 450 degrees Fahrenheit.

Add 1 tablespoon of oil and carrots into a large bowl. Stir the carrots around so they become coated with the oil.

Using oven mitts, remove the baking pans and distribute the carrots onto them.

Place the pans back into the oven and turn your timer on for 20 minutes or until the carrots become tender.

Take the carrots out of the oven.

Turn your oven to broiler mode.

Set a large stockpot on your stove and turn the range to medium-high.

Pour in the remaining olive oil and the onion. Let it cook for 5 minutes while stirring occasionally.

Pour in the broth, thyme, water, crushed red pepper, and sea salt. Stir well.

Let the mixture cook until the ingredients come to a boil.

Once the carrots are done in the oven, add them to the pot.

Remove the pot from the heat and carefully pour the soup into a blender. You will want to pour it in batches and remember to hold the lid of the blender with a rag and release the steam after 30 seconds, so it doesn't explode.

Once all the soup is mixed, add it all back into the pot and turn the range heat to medium. Cook until the soup is warm again.

Spread a piece of parchment paper on top of a baking sheet, set the four pieces of bread on the paper.

Sprinkle cheese across the slices and set them on the top rack in your oven.

Turn your oven to broil and let the slices of bread roast for a couple of minutes. Once the cheese is melted, remove the bread from the oven so they don't burn.

Chop the bread into croutons.

Divide the soup into serving bowls, add the croutons, and enjoy!

Nutrition Info: calories: 272, fats: 10 grams, carbohydrates: 38 grams, protein: 10 grams.

Greek Baked Cod

Servings: 4

Cooking Time: 12 Minutes

Ingredients:

1 ½ lb Cod fillet pieces (4–6 pieces)

5 garlic cloves, peeled and minced

1/4 cup chopped fresh parsley leaves

Lemon Juice Mixture:

5 tbsp fresh lemon juice

5 tbsp extra virgin olive oil

2 tbsp melted vegan butter

For Coating:

1/3 cup all-purpose flour

1 tsp ground coriander

3/4 tsp sweet Spanish paprika

3/4 tsp ground cumin

3/4 tsp salt

1/2 tsp black pepper

Directions:

Preheat oven to 400 degrees F

In a bowl, mix together lemon juice, olive oil, and melted butter, set aside

In another shallow bowl, mix all-purpose flour, spices, salt and pepper, set next to the lemon bowl to create a station

Pat the fish fillet dry, then dip the fish in the lemon juice mixture then dip it in the flour mixture, shake off excess flour

In a cast iron skillet over medium-high heat, add 2 tbsp olive oil

Once heated, add in the fish and sear on each side for color, but do not fully cook (just couple minutes on each side), remove from heat

With the remaining lemon juice mixture, add the minced garlic and mix

Drizzle all over the fish fillets

Bake for 10 minutes, for until the it begins to flake easily with a fork

allow the dish to cool completely

Distribute among the containers, store for 2-3 days

To Serve: Reheat in the microwave for 1-2 minutes or until heated through. Sprinkle chopped parsley. Enjoy!

Nutrition Info: Calories:321;Carbs: 16g;Total Fat: 18g;Protein: 23g

Pistachio Sole Fish

Servings: 4

Cooking Time: 10 Minutes

Ingredients:

4 (5 ounces boneless sole fillets

Salt and pepper as needed

½ cup pistachios, finely chopped

Zest of 1 lemon

Juice of 1 lemon

1 teaspoon extra virgin olive oil

Directions:

Pre-heat your oven to 350 degrees Fahrenheit

Line a baking sheet with parchment paper and keep it on the side

Pat fish dry with kitchen towels and lightly season with salt and pepper

Take a small bowl and stir in pistachios and lemon zest

Place sol on the prepped sheet and press 2 tablespoons of pistachio mixture on top of each fillet

Drizzle fish with lemon juice and olive oil

Bake for 10 minutes until the top is golden and fish flakes with a fork

Serve and enjoy!

Meal Prep/Storage Options: Store in airtight containers in your fridge for 1-2 days.

Nutrition Info: Calories: 166;Fat: 6g;Carbohydrates: 2g;Protein: 26g

Beef Tomato Soup

Servings: 6

Cooking Time: 1 Hour

Ingredients:

1 pound lean ground beef

1 medium onion, chopped

1 large green pepper, chopped

2 minced garlic cloves

1 large tomato, chopped

2 tablespoons tomato paste

2 tablespoons all-purpose flour

¼ cup uncooked rice

2 tablespoons fresh chopped parsley (additional for garnish)

4 cups beef broth

2 tablespoons olive oil

salt

pepper

Directions:

Add oil to large pot and heat over medium heat.

Add flour and keep whisking until thick paste forms.

Keep whisking for 4 minutes while it bubbles and begins to thin.

Add onions and sauté for 3-minutes.

Stir in tomato paste and ground beef, breaking up ground beef with a wooden spoon.

Cook for about 5 minutes.

Add garlic, peppers, and tomatoes.

Mix well until thoroughly combined.

Add broth and bring the mixture to a light boil.

Reduce heat to low, cover, and simmer for 30 minutes, making sure to stir from time to time.

Add rice and parsley and cook for another 15 minutes.

Once the soup has achieved its desired consistency, serve with a garnish of parsley.

This soup is best enjoyed with some crispy bread or boiled potatoes.

Nutrition Info: Calories: 268, Total Fat: 10.6 g, Saturated Fat: 2.8 g, Cholesterol: 68 mg, Sodium: 568 mg, Total Carbohydrate: 3 g, Dietary Fiber: 1.7 g, Total Sugars: 3.4 g, Protein: 28 g, Vitamin D: 0 mcg, Calcium: 25 mg, Iron: 15 mg, Potassium: 665 mg

Baked Tilapia

Servings: 4

Cooking Time: 15 Minutes

Ingredients:

1 lb tilapia fillets (about 8 fillets)

1 tsp olive oil

1 tbsp vegan butter

2 shallots finely chopped

3 garlic cloves minced

1 1/2 tsp ground cumin

1 1/2 tsp paprika

1/4 cup capers

1/4 cup fresh dill finely chopped

Juice from 1 lemon

Salt & Pepper to taste

Directions:

Preheat oven to 375 degrces F

Line a rimmed baking sheet with parchment paper or foil

Lightly mist with cooking spray, arrange the fish fillets evenly on baking sheet

In a small bowl, combine the cumin, paprika, salt and pepper

Season both sides of the fish fillets with the spice mixture

In a small bowl, whisk together the melted butter, lemon juice, shallots, olive oil, and garlic, and brush evenly over fish fillets

Top with the capers

Bake in the oven for 10-15 minutes, until cook through, but not overcooked

Remove from oven and allow the dish to cool completely

Distribute among the containers, store for 2-3 days

To Serve: Reheat in the microwave for 1-2 minutes or until heated through. Top with fresh dill. Serve!

Nutrition Info: Calories:;Total Fat: 5g;Protein: 21g

Herbal Lamb Cutlets With Roasted Veggies

Servings: 6

Cooking Time: 45 Minutes

Ingredients:

2 deseeded peppers, cut up into chunks

1 large sweet potato, peeled and chopped

2 sliced courgettes

1 red onion, cut into wedges

1 tablespoon olive oil

8 lean lamb cutlets

1 tablespoon thyme leaf, chopped

2 tablespoons mint leaves, chopped

Directions:

Preheat oven to 390degrees F.

In a large baking dish, place peppers, courgettes, sweet potatoes, and onion.

Drizzle all with oil and season with ground pepper.

Roast for about 25 minutes

Trim as much fat off the lamb as possible.

Mix in herbs with a few twists of ground black pepper.

Take the veggies out of the oven and push to one side of a baking dish.

Place lamb cutlets on another side, return to oven, and roast for another 10 minutes.

Turn the cutlets over, cook for another 10 minutes, and until the veggies are ready (lightly charred and tender).

Mix everything on the tray and spread over containers.

Nutrition Info: Calories: 268, Total Fat: 9.2 g, Saturated Fat: 3 g, Cholesterol: 100 mg, Sodium: mg, Total Carbohydrate: 10.7 g, Dietary Fiber: 2.4 g, Total Sugars: 4.1 g, Protein: 32.4 g, Vitamin D: 0 mcg, Calcium: 20 mg, Iron: 4 mg, Potassium: 365 mg

A Great Mediterranean Snapper

Servings: 2

Cooking Time: 10 Minutes

Ingredients:

2 tablespoons extra virgin olive oil

1 medium onion, chopped

2 garlic cloves, minced

1 teaspoon oregano

1 can (14 ounces tomatoes, diced with juice

½ cup black olives, sliced

4 red snapper fillets (each 4 ounce

Salt and pepper as needed

Garnish

¼ cup feta cheese, crumbled

¼ cup parsley, minced

Directions:

Pre-heat your oven to a temperature of 425-degree Fahrenheit

Take a 13x9 inch baking dish and grease it up with non-stick cooking spray

Take a large sized skillet and place it over medium heat

Add oil and heat it up

Add onion, oregano and garlic

Saute for 2 minutes

Add diced tomatoes with juice alongside black olives

Bring the mix to a boil

Remove the heat

Place the fish on the prepped baking dish

Season both sides with salt and pepper

Spoon the tomato mix over the fish

Bake for 10 minutes

Remove the oven and sprinkle a bit of parsley and feta

Enjoy!

Meal Prep/Storage Options: Store in airtight containers in your fridge for 1-3 days.

Nutrition Info: Calories: 269; Fat: 13g; Carbohydrates: 10g;Protein: 27g

Mediterranean Snapper

Servings: 4

Cooking Time: 12 Minutes

Ingredients:

non-stick cooking spray

2 tablespoons extra virgin olive oil

1 medium onion, chopped

2 garlic cloves, minced

1 teaspoon oregano

1 14-ounce can diced tomatoes, undrained

½ cup black olives, sliced

4 4-ounce red snapper fillets

salt

pepper

¼ cup crumbled feta cheese

¼ cup fresh parsley, minced

Directions:

Preheat oven to 425 degrees Fahrenheit.

Grease a 13x9 baking dish with non-stick cooking spray.

Heat oil in a large skillet over medium heat.

Add onion, oregano, garlic, and sauté for 2 minutes.

Add can of tomatoes and olives, and bring mixture to a boil; remove from heat.

Season both sides of fillets with salt and pepper and place in the baking dish.

Spoon the tomato mixture evenly over the fish.

Bake for 10 minutes.

Remove from oven and sprinkle with parsley and feta.

Enjoy!

Nutrition Info: Calories: 257, Total Fat: g, Saturated Fat: 1.7 g, Cholesterol: 53 mg, Sodium: 217 mg, Total Carbohydrate: 8.2 g, Dietary Fiber: 2.5 g, Total Sugars: 3.8 g, Protein: 31.3 g, Vitamin D: 0 mcg, Calcium: 85 mg, Iron: 1 mg, Potassium: 881 mg

Italian Skillet Chicken With Mushrooms And Tomatoes

Servings: 4

Cooking Time: 20 Minutes

Ingredients:

4 large chicken cutlets, boneless skinless chicken breasts cut into 1/4-inch thin cutlets

1 tbsp dried oregano, divided

1/2 cup all-purpose flour, more for later

8 oz Baby Bella mushrooms, cleaned, trimmed, and sliced

14 oz grape tomatoes, halved

2 tbsp chopped fresh garlic

Extra Virgin Olive Oil

1/2 cup white wine

1 tbsp freshly squeezed lemon juice, juice of 1/2 lemon

1 tsp salt, divided

1 tsp black pepper, divided

3/4 cup chicken broth

Handful baby spinach, optional

Directions:

Pat the chicken cutlets dry, season both sides with 2 tsp salt, 1/2 tsp black pepper, 1/2 tbsp dried oregano,

Coat the chicken cutlets with the flour, gently dust-off excess and set aside

In a large cast iron skillet with a lid, heat 2 tbsp olive oil

Once heated, brown the chicken cutlets on both sides, for about 3 minutes, then transfer the chicken cutlets to plate

In the same skillet, add more olive oil if needed,

Once heated, add in the mushrooms and sauté on medium-high for about 1 minute

Then add the tomatoes, garlic, the remaining 1/2 tbsp oregano, 1/2 tsp salt, and 1/2 tsp pepper, and 2 tsp flour, cook for 3 minutes or so, stirring regularly

Add in the white wine, cook briefly to reduce, then add the lemon juice and chicken broth

Bring the liquid to a boil, then transfer the chicken back into the skillet, cook over high heat for 3-4 minutes, then reduce the heat to medium-low, cover and cook for another 8 minutes or until the chicken is cooked through

Allow the dish to cool completely

Distribute among the containers, store for 3 days

To Serve: Reheat in the microwave for 1-2 minutes or until heated through. Serve with baby spinach, your favorite small pasta and a crusty Italian bread!

Nutrition Info: Calories:218;Carbs: 16g;Total Fat: 6g;Protein: 23g

Red Wine–braised Pot Roast With Carrots And Mushrooms

Servings: 4

Cooking Time: 25 Minutes

Ingredients:

1 pound tri-tip roast

¼ teaspoon kosher salt

1 tablespoon olive oil

2 cups chopped onion

1 teaspoon chopped garlic

3 medium carrots, cut into ½-inch pieces (2 cups)

2 large celery stalks, cut into ½-inch pieces (1 cup)

8 ounces button or cremini mushrooms, halved

½ teaspoon fennel seed

½ teaspoon dried thyme

½ teaspoon dried oregano

1 (14.5-ounce) can no-salt-added diced tomatoes

1 cup dry red wine, such as red zinfandel or cabernet sauvignon

1 cup reduced-sodium beef broth

Directions:

Preheat the oven to 325°F.

Season the roast with the salt.

Heat the oil in a Dutch oven or heavy-bottomed soup pot over high heat. Once the oil is hot, add the roast and brown for minutes on each side. Remove the roast to a plate.

Add the onion, garlic, carrots, celery, and mushrooms to the pot and cook for 5 minutes.

Add the fennel seed, thyme, oregano, tomatoes, red wine, and broth and bring to a simmer. Cover the pot with a tight-fitting lid or foil and place in the oven. Cook until the meat is very tender, about 3 hours.

Remove the roast to a plate and spoon the vegetables into a bowl with a slotted spoon. Place the pot on high heat and reduce the liquid by half, about 10 minutes. If your pot is extra wide, it will take less time for the liquid to reduce. Add more salt if needed.

After the meat has cooled, cut 12 slices against the grain. Place 3 slices, ¾ cup of vegetables, and ⅓ cup of sauce in each of 4 containers.

STORAGE: Store covered containers in the refrigerator for up to 5 days.

Nutrition Info: Total calories: 366; Total fat: 14g; Saturated fat: 4g; Sodium: 468mg; Carbohydrates: 23g; Fiber: 6g; Protein: 28g

Zoodles With Turkey Meatballs

Servings: 4-6

Cooking Time: 30 Minutes

Ingredients:

2 lbs (3 medium-sized) zucchini, spiralized

2 cups marinara sauce, store-bought

1/4 cup freshly grated Parmesan cheese

2 tsp salt

For The Meatballs:

1 ½ lbs ground turkey

1/2 cup Panko

1/4 cup freshly grated Parmesan cheese

2 large egg yolks

1 tsp dried oregano

1 tsp dried basil

1/2 tsp dried parsley

1/4 tsp garlic powder

1/4 tsp crushed red pepper flakes

Kosher salt, to taste

Freshly ground black pepper, to taste

Directions:

Preheat oven to 400 degrees F

Lightly oil a 9×13 baking dish or spray with nonstick spray

In a large bowl, combine the ground turkey, egg yolks, oregano, basil, Panko, Parmesan, parsley, garlic powder and red pepper flakes, season the mixture with salt and pepper, to taste

Use a wooden spoon or clean hands, stir well to combined

Roll the mixture into 1 1/2-to-2-inch meatballs, forming about 24 meatballs

Place the meatballs onto the prepared baking dish

Bake for 18-20 minutes, or until browned and the meatballs are cooked through, set aside

Place the zucchini in a colander over the sink, add the salt and gently toss to combine, allow to sit for 10 minutes

In a large pot of boiling water, cook zucchini for 30 seconds to 1 minute, drain well

Allow to cool, then distribute the zucchini into the containers, top with the meatballs, marinara sauce and the Parmesan. Store in the fridge for up to 4 days

To Serve: Reheat in the microwave for 1-2 minutes or until heated through and enjoy!

Nutrition Info: Calories:279;Total Fat: 13g;Total Carbs: ;Fiber: 3g;Protein: 31g

Italian Platter

Servings: 2

Cooking Time: 45 Minutes

Ingredients:

1 garlic clove, minced

5-ounce fresh button mushrooms, sliced

1/8 cup unsalted butter

¼ teaspoon dried thyme

1/3 cup heavy whipping cream

Salt and black pepper, to taste

2 (6-ounce grass-fed New York strip steaks

Directions:

Preheat the grill to medium heat and grease it.

Season the steaks with salt and black pepper, and transfer to the grill.

Grill steaks for about 10 minutes on each side and dish out in a platter.

Put butter, mushrooms, salt and black pepper in a pan and cook for about 10 minutes.

Add thyme and garlic and thyme and sauté for about 1 minute.

Stir in the cream and let it simmer for about 5 minutes.

Top the steaks with mushroom sauce and serve hot immediately.

Meal Prep Tip: You can store the mushroom sauce in refrigerator for about 2 days. Season the steaks carefully with salt and black pepper to avoid low or high quantities.

Nutrition Info: Calories: 332 ; Carbohydrates: 3.2g;Protein: 41.8g;Fat: 20.5g ;Sugar: 1.3g;Sodium: 181mg

Mediterranean Pizza

Servings: 4 To 8

Cooking Time: 20 Minutes

Ingredients:

1/2 cup artichoke hearts

Whole-wheat premade pizza crust

1 cup pesto sauce

1 cup spinach leaves

3 to 4 ounces of feta cheese

1 cup sun-dried tomatoes

3 ounces of mozzarella cheese

½ cup of olives

Olive oil

½ cup bell peppers

Chopped chicken, pepperoni, or salami

Directions:

Turn the temperature of your oven to 350 degrees Fahrenheit.

Use olive oil to brush the top of the whole wheat pizza crust.

Brush the pesto sauce on the pizza crust.

Top with all of the ingredients. You can start with the cheese or mix the ingredients in any way you wish. You can even get a little creative and have fun.

Set your pizza on a pizza pan or directly on your oven rack.

Set your timer to 10 minutes, but watch the pizza carefully so you do not burn the cheese.

Remove the pizza and let it cool down for a couple of minutes, then enjoy!

Nutrition Info: calories: 300, fats: 11 grams, carbohydrates: 29 grams, protein: 14 grams.

Roasted Vegetable Quinoa Bowl

Servings: 2

Cooking Time: 20 Minutes

Ingredients:

Quinoa:

¾ cup quinoa, rinsed

1 ½ cups

vegetable broth

Chili-Lime Kale

1/2 tsp chili powder

pinch salt

pinch pepper

2 cups packed kale, de-stemmed and chopped

1 tsp olive, coconut or canola oil

Juice of 1/4 lime

Garlic Roasted Broccoli:

2 cups broccoli,

2 tsp olive or canola oil

2 cloves garlic, minced

Pinch of salt

Black pepper

Curry Roasted Sweet Potatoes:

1 small sweet potato

1 tsp olive or canola oil

1 tsp curry powder

1 tsp sriracha

Pinch salt

Spicy Roasted Chickpeas:

1 ½ cups (cooked) chickpeas

1 tsp olive or canola oil

2 tsp sriracha

2 tsp soy sauce

Optional:

Lime

Avocado

Hummus

Red pepper flakes

Guacamole

Directions:

Preheat the oven to 400-degree F

Line a large baking sheet with parchment paper

Prepare the vegetables by chopping the broccoli into medium sized florets, de-stemming and chopping the kale, scrubbing and slicing the sweet potato into ¼" wide rounds

Take the broccoli florets and massage with oil, garlic, salt and pepper - making sure to work the ingredients into the tops of each florets - Place the florets in a row down in the center third of a large baking sheet

Using the same bowl, the broccoli in, mix together the chickpeas, oil, sriracha and soy sauce, then spread them out in a row next to the broccoli

In the same bowl combine the oil, curry powder, salt, and sriracha, add the sliced sweet potato and toss to coat, then lay the rounds on the remaining third of the baking tray

Bake for 10 minutes, flip the sweet potatoes and broccoli, and redistribute the chickpeas to cook evenly

Bake for another 8-12 minutes

For the Quinoa: Prepare the quinoa by rinsing and draining it. Add the rinsed quinoa and vegetable broth to a small saucepan and bring to a boil over high heat. Turn the heat down to medium-low, cover and allow to simmer for about 15 minutes. Once cooked, fluff with a fork and set aside

In the meantime, place a large skillet with 1 tsp oil, add in the kale and cook for about 5 minutes, or until nearly tender

Add in the salt, chili powder, and lime juice, toss to coat and cook for another 2-3 minutes

Allow all the ingredient to cool

Distribute among the containers – Add ½ to 1 cup of quinoa into each bowl, top with ½ of the broccoli, ½ kale, ½ the chickpeas and ½ sweet potatoes

To Serve: Reheat in the microwave for 1-2 minutes or until heated through. Enjoy

Nutrition Info: Calories:611;Carbs: 93g;Total Fat: 17g;Protein: 24g

Mediterranean Salmon

Servings: 4

Cooking Time: 15 Minutes

Ingredients:

½ cup of olive oil

¼ cup balsamic vinegar

4 garlic cloves, pressed

4 pieces salmon fillets

1 tablespoon fresh cilantro, chopped

1 tablespoon fresh basil, chopped

1½ teaspoons garlic salt

Directions:

Combine olive oil and balsamic vinegar.

Add salmon fillets to a shallow baking dish.

Rub the garlic onto the fillets.

Pour vinegar and oil all over, making sure to turn them once to coat them.

Season with cilantro, garlic salt, and basil.

Set aside and allow to marinate for about 10 minutes.

Preheat the broiler to your oven.

Place the baking dish with the salmon about 6 inches from the heat source.

Broil for 15 minutes until both sides are evenly browned and can be flaked with a fork.

Make sure to keep brushing with sauce from the pan.

Enjoy!

Nutrition Info: Calories: 459, Total Fat: 36.2 g, Saturated Fat: 5.2 g, Cholesterol: 78 mg, Sodium: 80 mg, Total Carbohydrate: 1.2 g, Dietary Fiber: 0.1 g, Total Sugars: 0.1 g, Protein: 34.8 g, Vitamin D: 0 mcg, Calcium: 71 mg, Iron: 1 mg, Potassium: 710 mg

Heartthrob Mediterranean Tilapia

Servings: 4

Cooking Time: 15 Minutes

Ingredients:

3 tablespoons sun-dried tomatoes, packed in oil, drained and chopped

1 tablespoon capers, drained

2 tilapia fillets

1 tablespoon oil from sun-dried tomatoes

1 tablespoon lemon juice

2 tablespoons kalamata olives, chopped and pitted

Directions:

Pre-heat your oven to 372-degree Fahrenheit

Take a small sized bowl and add sun-dried tomatoes, olives, capers and stir well

Keep the mixture on the side

Take a baking sheet and transfer the tilapia fillets and arrange them side by side

Drizzle olive oil all over them

Drizzle lemon juice

Bake in your oven for 10-15 minutes

After 10 minutes, check the fish for a "Flaky" texture

Once cooked properly, top the fish with tomato mix and serve!

Meal Prep/Storage Options: Store in airtight containers in your fridge for 1-3 days.

Nutrition Info: Calories: 183;Fat: 8g;Carbohydrates: 18g;Protein:183g

Garlic And Cajun Shrimp Bowl With Noodles

Servings: 2
Cooking Time: 15 Minutes

Ingredients:

1 sliced onion

1 tablespoon almond butter, but you can use regular butter as well

1 teaspoon onion powder

½ teaspoon salt

1 sliced red pepper

3 cloves of minced garlic

1 teaspoon paprika

20 jumbo shrimp, deveined and shells removed

3 tablespoons of ghee

2 zucchini, 3 if they are smaller in size, cut into noodles

Red pepper flakes and cayenne pepper, as desired

Directions:

In a small bowl, mix the pepper flakes, paprika, onion powder, salt, and cayenne pepper.

Toss the shrimp into the cajun mixture and coat the seafood thoroughly.

Add the ghee to a medium or large skillet and place on medium-low heat.

Once the ghee is melted, add the garlic and saute for minutes.

Carefully add the shrimp into the skillet and cook until they are opaque. Set the pan aside.

In a new pan, add the butter and allow it to melt.

Combine the zucchini noodles and cook on medium-low heat for 3 to 4 minutes.

Turn off the heat and place the zucchini noodles on serving dishes. Add the shrimp to the top and enjoy.

Nutrition Info: calories: 712, fats: 30 grams, carbohydrates: 20.1 grams, protein: grams.

Garlic Marinated Chicken

Servings: 3

Cooking Time: 15 Minutes

Ingredients:

1 ½ lbs. boneless skinless chicken breasts,

1/4 cup olive oil

1/4 cup lemon juice

3 cloves garlic, minced

1/2 tbsp dried oregano

1/2 tsp salt

Freshly cracked pepper

To Serve:

Rice or cauliflower rice

Roasted vegetables, such as carrots, asparagus, or green beans

Directions:

In a large Ziplock bag or dish, add in the olive oil, lemon juice, garlic, oregano, salt, and pepper

Close the bag and shake the ingredients to combine, or stir the ingredients in the dish until well combined

Filet each chicken breast into two thinner pieces and place the pieces in the bag or dish - make sure the chicken is completely covered in marinade and allow to marinate for up to minutes up to 8 hours, turn occasionally to maximize the marinade flavors

Once ready, heat a large skillet over medium heat

Once heated, transfer the chicken from the marinade to the hot skillet and cook on each side cooked through, about 7 minutes each side, depending on the size - Discard of any excess marinade

Transfer the cooked chicken from the skillet to a clean cutting board, allow to rest for five minutes before slicing

Distribute the chicken, cooked rice and vegetables among the containers. Store in the fridge for up to 4 days.

To Serve: Reheat in the microwave for 1-2 minutes or until heated through and enjoy!

Nutrition Info: Calories:446;Total Fat: 24g;Total Carbs: 4g;Fiber: 0g;Protein: 52g

Tabouli Salad

Servings: 6

Cooking Time: 30 Minutes

Ingredients:

½ cup extra fine bulgar wheat

4 firm Roma tomatoes, finely chopped, juice drained

1 English cucumber, finely chopped

2 bunches fresh parsley, stems removed, finely chopped

12-15 fresh mint leaves, finely chopped

4 green onions, finely chopped (white and green)

salt

3-4 tablespoons lime juice

3-4 tablespoons extra virgin olive oil

Romaine lettuce leaves

pita bread

Directions:

Wash bulgur wheat thoroughly and allow it to soak under water for 5 minutes.

Drain bulgur wheat well and set aside.

Add all vegetables, green onions, and herbs to a dish.

Add bulgur and season the mixture with salt.

Add limejuice and olive oil. Mix well.

Put to the jars and refrigerate.

Transfer to a serving platter and serve with sides of pita and romaine lettuce.

Nutrition Info: Calories: 136, Total Fat: 7.6 g, Saturated Fat: 1.1 g, Cholesterol: 0 mg, Sodium: 72 mg, Total Carbohydrate: 15.6 g, Dietary Fiber: 3.7 g, Total Sugars: 3.6 g, Protein: 3.4 g, Vitamin D: 0 mcg, Calcium: 71 mg, Iron: 3 mg, Potassium: 439 mg

Mediterranean Flounder

Servings: 4

Cooking Time: 45 Minutes

Ingredients:

Roma or plum tomatoes (5)

Extra-virgin olive oil (2 tbsp.)

Spanish onion (half of 1)

Garlic (2 cloves)

Italian seasoning (1 pinch)

Kalamata olives (24)

White wine (.25 cup)

Capers (.25 cup)

Lemon juice (1 tsp.)

Chopped basil (6 leaves)

Freshly grated parmesan cheese (3 tbsp.)

Flounder fillets (1 lb.)

Freshly torn basil (6 leaves)

Directions:

Set the oven to reach 425° Fahrenheit. Remove the pit and chop the olives (set aside.

Pour water into a saucepan and bring to boiling. Plunge the tomatoes into the water and remove immediately.

Add to a dish of ice water and drain. Remove the skins, chop, and set to the side for now.

Heat a skillet with the oil using the medium temperature heat setting. Chop and toss in the onions. Sauté them for around four minutes.

Dice and add the garlic, tomatoes, and seasoning. Simmer for five to seven minutes.

Stir in the capers, wine, olives, half of the basil, and freshly squeezed lemon juice.

Lower the heat setting and blend in the cheese. Simmer it until the sauce is thickened (15 min..

Arrange the flounder into a shallow baking tin. Add the sauce and garnish with the remainder of the basil leaves.

Set the timer to bake it for 12 minutes until the fish is easily flaked.

Nutrition Info: Calories: 282;Protein: 24.4 grams; Fat: 15.4 grams

Greek Lemon Chicken Soup

Servings: 8

Cooking Time: 20 Minutes

Ingredients:

10 cups chicken broth

3 tbsp olive oil

8 cloves garlic, minced

1 sweet onion

1 large lemon, zested

2 boneless skinless chicken breasts

1 cup Israeli couscous (pearl)

1/2 tsp crushed red pepper

2 oz crumbled feta

1/3 cup chopped chive

Salt, to taste

Pepper, to taste

Directions:

In a large 6-8-quart sauce pot over medium-low heat, add the olive oil

Once heated, sauté the onion and minced the garlic for 3-4 minutes to soften

Then add in the chicken broth, raw chicken breasts, lemon zest, and crushed red pepper to the pot Raise the heat to high, cover, and bring to a boil

Once boiling, reduce the heat to medium, then simmer for 5 minutes

Stir in the couscous, 1 tsp salt, and black pepper to taste

Simmer another 5 minute, then turn the heat off

Using tongs, remove the two chicken breasts from the pot and transfer to a plate

Use a fork and the tongs to shred the chicken, then return to the pot

Stir in the crumbled feta cheese and chopped chive

Season to taste with salt and pepper as needed

Allow the soup to cool completely

Distribute among the containers, store for 2-3 days

To Serve: Reheat in the microwave for 1-2 minutes or until heated through, or reheat on the stove

Nutrition Info: Calories:2Carbs: 23g;Total Fat: g; Protein: 11g

Mediterranean Steamed Salmon With Fresh Herbs And Lemon

Servings: 4

Cooking Time: 15 Minutes

Ingredients:

1 yellow onion, halved and sliced

4 green onions spring onions, trimmed and sliced lengthwise, divided

1 lb skin-on salmon fillet (such as wild Alaskan), cut into 4 portions

1/2 tsp Aleppo pepper

4 to 5 garlic cloves, chopped

Extra virgin olive oil

A large handful fresh parsley

1 lemon, thinly sliced

1 tsp ground coriander

1 tsp ground cumin

1/2 cup white wine (or you can use water or low-sodium broth, if you prefer)

Kosher salt, to taste

Black pepper, to taste

Directions:

Prepare a large piece of wax paper or parchment paper (about 2 feet long) and place it right in the center of a - inch deep pan or braiser

Place the sliced yellow onions and a sprinkle a little bit of green onions the onions on the bottom of the braiser

Arrange the salmon, skin-side down, on top, season with kosher salt and black pepper

In a small bowl, mix together the coriander, cumin, and Aleppo pepper, coat top of salmon with the spice mixture, and drizzle with a little bit of extra virgin olive oil

Then add garlic, parsley and the remaining green onions on top of the salmon (make sure that everything is arrange evenly over the salmon portions.)

Arrange the lemon slices on top of the salmon

Add another drizzle of extra virgin olive oil, then add the white wine

Fold the parchment paper over to cover salmon, secure the edges and cover the braiser with the lid

Place the braising pan over medium-high heat, cook for 5 minutes

Lower the heat to medium, cook for another 8 minutes, covered still

Remove from heat and allow to rest undisturbed for about 5 minutes.

Remove the lid and allow the salmon to cool completely

Distribute among the containers, store for 2-3 days

To Serve: Reheat in the microwave for 1-2 minutes or until heated through.

Recipe Notes: The pan or braiser you use needs to have a lid to allow the steamed salmon.

Nutrition Info: Calories:321;Carbs: g;Total Fat: 18g;Protein: 28g

Grilled Salmon Tzatziki Bowl

Servings: 2

Cooking Time: 15 Minutes

Ingredients:

8–10 ounces salmon, serves 2

Olive oil for brushing

Salt and pepper

1 lemon- sliced in half

Tzatziki:

½ cup plain yogurt

½ cup sour cream

1 garlic clove- finely minced

1 tbsp lemon juice, more to taste

1 tbsp olive oil

½ tsp kosher salt

¼ tsp white pepper or black

⅛ cup fresh chopped dill (or mint, cilantro or Italian parsley – or a mix)

1 ½ cups finely sliced or diced cucumber

Optional Bowl Additions:

Cooked Quinoa or rice

Arugula or other greens

Grilled veggies like eggplant, peppers, tomatoes, or zucchini

Fresh veggies of your choice - radishes, cucumber, tomatoes, sprouts

Garnish with olive oil, lemon, and fresh herbs

Directions:

Preheat heat grill to medium high

Cook 1 cup quinoa or rice on the stove, according to directions, allow to cool

Brush the salmon with olive oil, season with salt and pepper, set aside

Create the Tzatziki, by adding plain yogurt, sour cream, garlic clove, lemon juice, olive oil, kosher salt, and white pepper in a bowl, taste and add more lemon juice if desired, store in fridge

Place the salmon on the grill, along with the veggies of you choose to grill, brushing all with olive oil, salt and pepper

Grill the salmon on both sides for 3-4 minutes, or until cooked through

Then grill the lemon, open side down, until good grill marks appear

Once the veggies and salmon are done, allow them to cool

Distribute among the containers - Divide quinoa among the containers, arrange the grilled vegetables and salmon over top.

To Serve: Reheat in the microwave for 1 minute or until heated through. Top with the greens and the fresh veggies, then drizzle a little olive oil on top and season with salt, squeeze the grilled lemon over the whole bowl, spoon the tzatziki over top the salmon, sprinkle with the fresh dill or other herbs. Enjoy with a glass of wine.

Nutrition Info: Calories:458;Carbs: 29g;Total Fat: 24g;Protein: 30g

Smoky Chickpea, Chard, And Butternut Squash Soup

Servings: 8

Cooking Time: 35 Minutes

Ingredients:

2 slices bacon (about 1 ounce), chopped

1 cup chopped onion

1 teaspoon chopped garlic

1 teaspoon smoked paprika

½ teaspoon kosher salt

2 teaspoons fresh thyme leaves, roughly chopped

1½ pounds butternut squash, peeled, seeded, and cut into 1-inch cubes

1 large bunch chard, stems and leaves chopped

2 (15.5-oz) cans low-sodium chickpeas, drained and rinsed

32 ounces low-sodium chicken broth

1 tablespoon freshly squeezed lemon juice

8 teaspoons grated Parmesan or Pecorino Romano cheese for garnish

Directions:

Place a soup pot, at least 4½ quarts in size, on the stove over medium heat. Add the chopped bacon and cook until the fat has rendered and the bacon is crisp. Remove the bacon pieces to a plate.

Add the chopped onion and garlic to the same pot. Sauté in the bacon fat until the onion is soft, about 5 minutes. Add the paprika, salt, and thyme. Stir to coat the onion well. Add the squash, chard, chickpeas, and broth to the pot.

Turn the heat to high, bring the soup to a boil, then turn the heat down to low and simmer until the squash is tender, about 20 minutes.

Add the lemon juice. If necessary, add another pinch of salt to taste.

Place 2 cups of cooled soup in each of 4 containers and top each serving with 2 teaspoons of cheese. Store the remaining 4 Servings: in the freezer to eat later.

STORAGE: Store covered containers in the refrigerator for up to 5 days. If frozen, soup will last 4 months.

Nutrition Info:: Total calories: 194; Total fat: 2g; Saturated fat: 1g; Sodium: 530mg; Carbohydrates: 34g; Fiber: 11g; Protein: 12g

Herbed Tuna Salad Wraps

Servings: 4

Cooking Time: 15 Minutes

Ingredients:

1 (11-ounce) pouch tuna in water

1 cup parsley leaves, chopped

¼ cup mint leaves, chopped

¼ cup minced shallot

1½ teaspoons sumac

1 teaspoon Dijon mustard

1 tablespoon olive oil

1 tablespoon freshly squeezed lemon juice

¼ cup unsalted sunflower seeds

16 large or medium romaine or bibb lettuce leaves

1 red bell pepper, cut into thin sticks (3 to 4 inches long)

3 Persian cucumbers, cut into thin sticks (3 to 4 inches long)

Directions:

In a large bowl, mix together the tuna, parsley, mint, shallot, sumac, mustard, oil, lemon juice, and sunflower seeds.

Place ¾ cup of tuna salad in each of 4 containers. Place 4 lettuce leaves, one quarter of the peppers, and one quarter of the cucumbers in each of 4 separate containers so that they don't get soggy from the tuna salad.

STORAGE: Store covered containers in the refrigerator for up to 4 days.

TIP Tuna in pouches is preferable to cans, because pouches don't need to be drained and the tuna isn't soggy. You can substitute canned salmon, canned sardines, or even shredded rotisserie chicken for the tuna in this salad.

Nutrition Info: Total calories: 223; Total fat: 9g; Saturated fat: 1g; Sodium: 422mg; Carbohydrates: 12g; Fiber: 4g; Protein: 24g

Mediterranean Potato Salad

Servings: 6

Cooking Time: 30 Minutes

Ingredients:

3 tablespoons extra virgin olive oil

½ cup of sliced olives

1 tablespoon olive juice

3 tablespoons lemon juice, freshly squeezed is best

2 tablespoons of mint, fresh and torn

¼ teaspoon sea salt

2 stalks of sliced celery

2 pounds baby potatoes

2 tablespoons of chopped oregano, fresh is best

Directions:

Cut the potatoes into inch cubes.

Toss the potatoes into a medium saucepan and cover them with water.

Place the saucepan on the stove over high heat.

Once the potatoes start to boil, bring the heat down to medium-low.

Let the potatoes simmer for 13 to 1minutes. When you poke the potatoes with a fork and they feel tender, they are done.

As the potatoes are simmering, grab a small bowl and mix the oil, olive juice, lemon juice, and salt. Whisk the ingredients together well.

Once the potatoes are done, drain them and pour the potatoes into a bowl.

Take the juice mixture and pour 3 tablespoons over the potatoes right away.

Combine the potatoes with the celery and olives.

Prior to serving, sprinkle the potatoes with the mint, oregano, and rest of the dressing.

Nutrition Info: calories: 175, fats: 7 grams, carbohydrates: 27 grams, protein: 3 grams.

Mediterranean Zucchini Noodles

Servings: 2

Cooking Time: 10 Minutes

Ingredients:

2 large zucchini or 1 package of store-bought zucchini noodles

1 tsp olive oil

4 cloves garlic diced

10 oz cherry tomatoes cut in half

2-4 oz plain hummus

1 tsp oregano

1/2 tsp red wine vinegar plus more to taste

1/2 cup jarred artichoke hearts, drained and chopped

1/4 cup sun-dried tomatoes, drained and chopped

Salt, to taste

Pepper to taste

Parmesan and fresh basil for topping

Directions:

Prepare the zucchini by cutting of the ends off zucchini and spiralize, set aside

In a pan over medium heat, add in olive oil

Then add in the garlic and cherry tomatoes to the pan, sauté until tomatoes begin to burst, about to 4 minutes

Add in the zucchini noodles, sun-dried tomatoes, hummus, oregano, artichoke hearts and red wine vinegar to the pan, sauté for 1-2 minutes, or until zucchini is tender-crisp and heated through

Season to taste with salt and pepper as needed

Allow the zoodle to cool

Distribute among the containers, store in the fridge for 2-3 days

To Serve: Reheat in the microwave for 30 seconds or until heated through, serve immediately with parmesan and fresh basil. Enjoy

Nutrition Info: Calories:241;Carbs: 8g;Total Fat: 37g;Protein: 10g

Lobster Salad

Servings: 2

Cooking Time: 15 Minutes

Ingredients:

¼ yellow onion, chopped

¼ yellow bell pepper, seeded and chopped

¾ pound cooked lobster meat, shredded

1 celery stalk, chopped

Black pepper, to taste

¼ cup avocado mayonnaise

Directions:

Mix together all the ingredients in a bowl and stir until well combined.

Refrigerate for about 3 hours and serve chilled.

Put the salad into a container for meal prepping and refrigerate for about 2 days.

Nutrition Info: Calories: 336 ;Carbohydrates: 2g;Protein: 27.2g;Fat: 25.2g ;Sugar: 1.2g;Sodium: 926mg

GREAT MEDITERRANEAN DIET RECIPES

Red lentil soup

Preparation time: 10 minutes

Cooking time: 45 minutes

Servings: 4

Ingredients:

Four minced garlic cloves

¼ cup olive oil

1 tsp curry powder

Two chopped carrots

2 tsp ground cumin

One chopped onion

½ tsp dried thyme

1 cup brown lentils

28 oz diced tomatoes

4 cups vegetable broth

1 tsp salt

2 cups of water

One pinch of red pepper flakes

1 cup chopped kale

Black pepper to taste

1.5 tbsp lemon juice

Directions : Cook carrots and onions in ¼ cup of heated olive oil in a Dutch oven over medium flame for five minutes.
Stir in thyme, cumin, garlic, and curry powder,
Cook for half a minute.
Add tomatoes and cook for another five minutes.
Add pepper flakes, broth, salt, lentils, black pepper, and water in a Dutch oven.
Let it boil. Cover the oven and lower the flame and let it simmer for 30 minutes.
Blend a portion of soup of about two cups in a food processor and transfer it into the pot again.
Mix chopped greens and cook for another five minutes.
Remove from the flame and mix lemon juice and serve.

Nutrition Info: Calories: 366 kcal Fat: 15.5 g Protein: 14.5 g Carbs: 47.8 g Fiber: 10.8 g

Salmon soup

Preparation time: 10 minutes
Cooking time: 12 minutes
Servings: 4

Ingredients:

Olive oil
½ chopped green bell pepper
Four chopped green onions
Four minced garlic cloves
5 cups chicken broth
1 oz chopped dill
1 lb sliced gold potatoes
1 tsp dry oregano
One sliced carrot
¾ tsp coriander
Kosher salt to taste
½ tsp cumin
Black pepper to taste
Zest of one lemon
1 lb sliced salmon fillet
1 tbsp lemon juice

Directions :

Cook onions, garlic, and bell pepper in heated olive oil in a pot over medium flame for four minutes.

Stir in the dill and cook for half a minute.

Pour broth into the pot. Add carrot, potatoes, salt, spices, and pepper.

Let it boil. Reduce the flame and let it simmer for six minutes.

Add salmon and cook for five more minutes.

Add lemon juice and zest and cook for one minute.

Serve the soup and enjoy it.

Nutrition Info: Calories: 338 kcal Fat: 10.7 g Protein: 32.4 g Carbs: 30.2 g Fiber: 4.1 g

Falafel sandwiches

Preparation time: 20 minutes
Cooking time: 10 minutes
Servings: 4 sandwiches

Ingredients:

4 Pita Breads

1 cup arugula

1 tbsp lemon

1/2 cup tahini sauce

12 falafels

One sliced red onion

1/2 cup tabbouleh salad

Three sprigs mint

Directions :

Spread tahini sauce followed by the addition of arugula and crushed falafels over pita bread. Add tabbouleh salad, mint, and onions over pita and drizzle lemon juice.
Wrap the pita bread and serve.

Nutrition Info: Calories: 360 kcal Fat: 17 g Protein: 12 g Carbs: 44 g Fiber: 4 g

Roasted tomato basil soup

Preparation time: 10 minutes
Cooking time: 50 minutes
Servings: 6

Ingredients:
3 lb halved Roma tomatoes
Olive oil
Two chopped carrots
Salt to taste
Two chopped yellow onions
Black pepper to taste
Five minced garlic cloves
2 oz basil leaves
1 cup crushed tomatoes
Three thyme sprigs
1 tsp dry oregano
2 tsp thyme leaves
½ tsp paprika
2.5 cups water
½ tsp cumin
1 tbsp lime juice

Directions :

Mix salt, olive oil, carrot, black pepper, and tomatoes in a bowl.

Transfer carrot mixture to a baking tray and bake in a preheated oven at 450 degrees for 30 minutes.

Blend baked tomato mixture in a blender. You can use a little water if needed during blending.

Sauté onions in heated olive oil over medium flame in a pot for three minutes.

Mix garlic and cook for one more minute.

Transfer the blended tomato mixture to the pot, followed by the addition of crushed tomatoes, water, spices, thyme, salt, basil, and pepper.

Let it boil. Reduce the flame and simmer for 20 minutes.

Drizzle lemon juice and serve.

Nutrition Info: Calories: 104 kcal Fat: 0.8 g Protein: 4.3 g Carbs: 23.4 g Fiber: 5.4 g

Greek black-eyed peas stew

Preparation time: 5 minutes

Cooking time: 55 minutes

Servings: 6

Ingredients:

Olive oil

Four chopped garlic cloves

30 oz black-eyed peas

One chopped yellow onion

One chopped green bell pepper

15 oz diced tomato

Three chopped carrots

1 tbsp of lime juice

2 cups of water

1.5 tsp cumin

One dry bay leaf

1 tsp dry oregano

Kosher salt to taste

½ tsp red pepper flakes

½ tsp paprika

Black pepper to taste

1 cup chopped parsley

Directions :

Cook garlic and onions in a heated oven in a Dutch oven over medium flame for five minutes with constant stirring.

Stir in tomatoes, pepper, water, spices, bay leaf, and salt.

Let it boil.

Mix black-eyed beans and cook for five more minutes.

Cover the oven and reduce the flame. Simmer for 30 minutes.

Squeeze lemon juice and mix.

Serve and enjoy.

Nutrition Info: Calories: 187 kcal Fat: 3.5 g Protein: 9.3 g Carbs: 33 g Fiber: 9.6 g

Juicy salmon burgers

Preparation time: 10 minutes
Cooking time: 4 minutes
Servings: 4

Ingredients:
1.5 lb sliced salmon fillet
3 tbsp minced green onions
1 tsp coriander
2 tsp Dijon mustard
1/3 cup bread crumbs
1 tsp sumac
1 cup chopped parsley
½ tsp sweet paprika
Kosher Salt to taste
¼ cup olive oil
½ tsp black pepper
One lemon
Toppings
One sliced red onion
Tzatziki Sauce
One sliced tomato
6 oz baby arugula

Directions :

Blend mustard and salmon in a blender.

Shift the mixture in a container. Add all the spices, parsley, salt, and onions. Mix well and set aside for 30 minutes.

Make patties out of salmon mixture and place in a tray.

Coat all the patties with bread crumbs from both sides.

Fry the patties in heated olive oil over medium flame for five minutes each from both sides.

Drizzle lemon juice over the cooked patties.

Spread Tzatziki sauce over the bun, followed by the layer of salmon, arugula, onions, and tomatoes. The salmon burgers are ready. Serve and enjoy it.

Nutrition Info: Calories: 365 kcal Fat: 19.5 g Protein: 40 g Carbs: 9.5 g Fiber: 1.6 g

Braised eggplant and chickpeas

Preparation time: 20 minutes

Cooking time: 55 minutes

Servings: 6

Ingredients:

1.5 lb chopped eggplant

Olive Oil

Kosher salt

One chopped yellow onion

One chopped carrot

One diced green bell pepper

Six minced garlic cloves

1.5 tsp sweet paprika

Two dry bay leaves

1 tsp organic coriander

¾ tsp cinnamon

1 tsp dry oregano

½ tsp organic turmeric

28 oz chopped tomato

½ tsp black pepper

30 oz chickpeas

Handful parsley and mint for garnishing

Directions :

Sauté onions, carrots, and bell peppers in heated olive oil over medium flame for four minutes with constant stirring.

Stir in salt, bay leaf, garlic, and spices and cook for one minute.

Mix eggplant, chickpeas, tomato, and chickpea liquid.

Let it boil for ten minutes.

Remove the pan from flame and cover.

Now, bake in a preheated oven at 400 degrees for 45 minutes.

Sprinkle herbs and serve with any sauce.

Nutrition Info: Calories: 240 kcal Fat: 5.1 g Protein: 10.6 g Carbs: 42 g Fiber: 15 g

Mediterranean tuna salad sandwiches

Preparation time: 5 minutes

Cooking time: 0 minute

Servings: 4

Ingredients:

4 tsp red wine vinegar

4 tsp olive oil

Eight bread slices

¼ cup chopped red onion

12 oz tuna

1/3 cup chopped sun-dried tomatoes

¼ tsp black pepper

¼ cup sliced olives

3 tbsp mayonnaise

2 tsp capers

Four lettuce leaves

Directions :

Mix wine and olive oil.

Brush bread from both sides with oil mixture.

Mix all the ingredients except lettuce and bread slices in a bowl.

Place lettuce on each bread slices brushed with oil. Spread tuna mixture and cover with second bread piece and serve.

Nutrition Info: Calories: 293 kcal Fat: 10 g Protein: 21.2 g Carbs: 31.3 g Fiber: 4.6 g

Moroccan vegetable tagine

Preparation time: 15 minutes

Cooking time: 40 minutes

Servings: 5

Ingredients:

¼ cup extra virgin olive oil

Ten chopped garlic cloves

Two chopped yellow onions

Two chopped carrots

One sliced sweet potato

Two sliced potatoes

Salt

1 tsp coriander

1 tbsp Harissa spice

1 tsp cinnamon

2 cups tomatoes

½ tsp turmeric

½ cup chopped dried apricot

2 cups cooked chickpeas

Handful fresh parsley leaves

½ cup vegetable broth

1 tbsp lemon juice

Directions :

Sauté onions in heated olive oil at high flame for five minutes in a Dutch oven.

Stir in veggies, salt, garlic, and spices. Mix well and cook for eight minutes over medium flame with constant stirring.

Mix in broth, apricot, and tomatoes and cook for the next ten minutes.

Reduce the flame and let it simmer for 25 minutes.

Add chickpeas and cook for five minutes.

Sprinkle parsley and lemon juice and mix well.

Serve and enjoy it.

Nutrition Info: Calories: 448 kcal Fat: 18.4 g Protein: 16.9 g Carbs: 60.7 g Fiber: 24 g

Mediterranean grilled balsamic chicken with olive tapenade

Preparation time: 10 minutes
Cooking time: 30 minutes
Servings: 2

Ingredients:
Two boneless chicken breasts
1/4 cup olive oil
1/4 cup balsamic vinegar
1/8 cup garlic mustard
1.5 tbsp balsamic vinegar
Three minced garlic cloves
1 tbsp lemon juice
1 tbsp chopped herbs of choice
1 tsp kosher salt
1/2 tsp black pepper

Directions :
Combine garlic, balsamic vinegar, lemon juice, pepper, olive oil, herbs, salt, and mustard in a bowl. Add chicken and toss well to coat chicken.
Set aside for three hours.
Brush oil over chicken pieces and grill gates.

Cook chicken on grill gates for ten minutes from both sides.

Occasionally brush the chicken with marinade while grilling it.

When marks appear over the chicken, shift the chicken to the grill gate's cooler side and cook there for 12 minutes.

Again, shift the chicken to the heated side of the grill gate and cook for ten more minutes.

Place the grilled chicken on a plate and cover to keep it warm.

Serve and enjoy it.

Nutrition Info: Calories: 352 kcal Fat: 21 g Protein: 35 mg Carbs: 5 g Fiber: 1 g

Linguine and zucchini noodles with shrimp

Preparation time: 20 minutes

Cooking time: 20 minutes

Servings: 6

Ingredients:

2/3 cup extra virgin olive oil

1 lb shrimp

Four minced garlic cloves

Black pepper to taste

12 oz wheat linguine

kosher salt to taste

1/2 cup shredded Parmesan cheese

3 tbsp butter

Three zucchinis

One lemon zested

1 tsp red chili flakes

3 tbsp lemon juice

A handful of chopped parsley

Directions :

Add salt, garlic, shrimps, pepper, and olive oil. Toss well to coat evenly. Keep it aside.

Pour water into a pot and add salt to it. Let it boil and cook linguine in boiling water. Drain linguine and set aside.

Heat olive oil in a skillet over medium heat and cook shrimps in it for three minutes from both sides. Shift the cooked shrimps into the plate.

Melt butter in the same pan and sauté garlic, lemon juice, chili flakes, and lemon zest for one minute.

Pour in pasta water in another pan and cook for three minutes. Add zucchini noodles and cook for two minutes with constant stirring.

Transfer the noodles to the garlic mixture pan. Add linguine and cheese. Toss well.

Pour in more of the pasta water to make a sauce of the desired level.

Add shrimp, zucchini, salt, and pepper, and mix well.

You can spread more cheese if you like.

Garnish with parsley and serve.

Nutrition Info: Calories: 521 kcal Fat: 22 g Protein: 28 g Carbs: 52 g Fiber: 4 g

Chicken gyros with Tzatziki sauce

Preparation time: 10 minutes

Cooking time: 8 minutes

Servings: 4

Ingredients:

Greek Chicken

1 tbsp lemon juice

1/2 cup plain yogurt

1.25 tsp Mediterranean-spiced salt

2 tbsp extra-virgin olive oil

1 cup Tzatziki sauce

Four slices of pita bread

Four chopped tomatoes

1/4 sliced red onion

Tzatziki Sauce

½ halved cucumber

¾ cup Greek yogurt

Two minced garlic cloves

1 tbsp red wine vinegar

1 tbsp chopped dill

One pinch of kosher salt

One pinch of black pepper

Directions :

Marinate the chicken by mixing it with lemon juice, salt, and yogurt. Set aside for one hour.

Heat olive oil in a skillet over medium flame.

Add chicken without marinade and cook for five minutes from both sides. Transfer the cooked brown chicken to the plate.

Mix all the ingredients of Tzatziki sauce in a bowl and set aside. The Tzatziki sauce is ready.

Toast pita bread and place Tzatziki sauce, tomatoes, onions, and chicken pieces over pita bread. Wrap and serve.

Nutrition Info: Calories: 411 kcal Fat: 21 g Protein: 44 g Carbs: 10 g Fiber: 1 g

Greek chicken marinade

Preparation time: 5 minutes
Cooking time: 15 minutes
Servings: 4

Ingredients:
1 lb boneless chicken breasts
¼ cup olive oil
½ tsp black pepper
1/3 cup Greek yogurt
Four lemons
2 tbsp dried oregano
Five minced garlic cloves
1 tsp kosher salt

Directions : Mix all the ingredients in a bowl and set aside for three hours.
Preheat the grill and grill chicken and lemon slices for 20 minutes from both sides.
Slice the grilled chicken and serve.

Nutrition Info: Calories: 304 kcal Fat: 19 g Protein: 25 g Carbs: 14 g Fiber: 4 g

Mediterranean chicken quinoa bowl with broccoli and tomato

Preparation time: 10 minutes

Cooking time: 30 minutes

Servings: 3

Ingredients:

Chicken

6 oz boneless chicken breast

1 cup Easy Roasted Feta and Broccoli

1/2 cup olive oil

1/2 tsp kosher salt

Zest of one lemon

2 tsp dried oregano

1.5 tbsp lemon juice

1/4 tsp black pepper

Two minced garlic cloves

1/2 cup Easy Roasted Tomatoes

Quinoa

1 tsp kosher salt

1 cup dried quinoa

Feta cheese to taste

Directions :

Mix lemon juice, oregano, salt, olive oil, garlic, lemon zest, and pepper in a bowl.

Add chicken and toss well. Set aside for one hour.

Cook chicken in heat olive oil over medium flame for 15 minutes.

Lower the flame and stir in tomatoes and broccoli and cook. Set aside.

Add water and salt to a pot and bring it to a boil.

Add quinoa and cook for ten minutes.

Drain the quinoa and set aside.

Add quinoa in a bowl, followed by the addition of chicken and veggies. Sprinkle salt, cheese, oil, and pepper.

Serve and enjoy it.

Nutrition Info: Calories: 481 kcal Fat: 23 g Protein: 24 g Carbs: 45 g Fiber: 7 g

Chicken piccata

Preparation time: 10 minutes
Cooking time: 10 minutes
Servings: 4

Ingredients:

1.5 lb boneless chicken breasts
One lemon
2 tbsp canola oil
1 tsp kosher salt
1/3 cup all-purpose flour
1 cup chicken broth
1 tsp black pepper
2 tbsp capers
3 tbsp butter

Directions :

Mix salt, flour, and pepper in a bowl. Coat chicken with the flour mixture. Set aside.

Cook chicken pieces in heated butter and canola oil over medium flame for five minutes from both sides. Shift cooked pieces onto the plate.

Lower the flame and pour broth and add sliced lemon, butter (1 tbsp), lemon juice, capers, and cook for five minutes.

Pour the sauce over chicken pieces and serve with cauliflower or noodles.

Nutrition Info: Calories: 381 kcal Fat: 20 g Protein: 37 g Carbs: 11 g Fiber: 1 g

Chopped grilled vegetable with farro

Preparation time: 5 minutes

Cooking time: 50 minutes

Servings: 2

Ingredients: 1 cup dried farro

1 Portobello mushroom

3 cups vegetable broth

One sliced red bell pepper

1/2 sliced red onion

8 oz asparagus

One sliced zucchini

Olive oil as required

1/4 cup halved Kalamata olives

One sliced yellow squash

Kosher salt to taste

1-pint Greek yogurt

Black pepper to taste

2 tbsp minced cucumber

One chopped garlic clove

1 tbsp lemon juice

1 tsp chopped dill

1 tsp chopped mint

Red bell pepper hummus

1/8 cup feta cheese

Directions :

In a large pot, add broth and farro. Let it boil over a high flame.

Lower the flame to medium and cook for half an hour with occasional stirring.

Mix veggies with salt, olive oil, and pepper.

Grill the veggies in a preheated grill until marks appear on them. Keep them aside.

Whisk cucumber, salt, mint, dill, yogurt, lemon juice, and garlic in a bowl.

Make the layers of farro, grilled veggies, hummus, olives, and cheese.

Pour yogurt sauce and sprinkle mint and serve.

Nutrition Info: Calories: 140 kcal Fat: 6 g Protein: 4 g Carbs: 20 g Fiber: 5 g

30 minutes' pork scaloppini with lemons and capers

Preparation time: 10 minutes

Cooking time: 20 minutes

Servings: 4

Ingredients:

Four boneless pork chops

1/4 cup all-purpose flour

Eight sage leaves

kosher salt to taste

2 tbsp chopped parsley

4 tbsp butter

Black pepper to taste

1 tbsp vegetable oil

1/4 cup capers

1/2 cup white wine

1 cup chicken stock

One sliced lemon

4 tbsp lemon juice

Directions :

One each pork chops, place two sage leaves on both sides. Set aside.

In a bowl, whisk salt, flour, and pepper.

Coat pork chops with flour. Keep the sage leaves in place.

Melt butter in a skillet over medium flame.

Cook pork chops for five minutes from both sides.

Clean the skillet and melt butter in it.

Pour wine and add capers in skillet. Cook to concentrate the wine.

Pour stock, lemon slices, and lemon juice. Let it boil for five more minutes.

Place pork in sauce and cook for two minutes.

Sprinkle parsley and serve.

Nutrition Info: Calories: 415 kcal Fat: 7 g Protein: 31 g Carbs: 14 g Fiber: 8 g

Greek chicken kebabs

Preparation time: 40 minutes

Cooking time: 15 minutes

Servings: 6

Ingredients:

1 lb boneless chicken breasts

1/4 cup olive oil

One sliced red bell pepper

1/3 cup Greek yogurt

10 tbsp lemons juice

Four chopped garlic cloves

Zest of one lemon

2 tbsp dried oregano

1/2 tsp black pepper

One sliced zucchini

1 tsp kosher salt

One sliced red onion

Directions :

Whisk all the ingredients except chicken in a bowl. Add chicken and toss to coat chicken evenly. Set aside four hours for better results.

Thread chicken, zucchini, onion, and bell pepper on the skewers.

Grill the chicken, skewers on a preheated grill for 15 minutes, occasionally turning and basting with marinade.

Nutrition Info: Calories: 224 kcal Fat: 13 g Protein: 18 g Carbs: 13 g Fiber: 4 g

Shrimp pasta with roasted red peppers and artichokes

Preparation time: 10 minutes

Cooking time: 25 minutes

Servings: 8

Ingredients:

12 oz farfalle pasta

1/4 cup butter

1.5 lb shrimp

Three chopped garlic cloves

1 cup sliced artichoke hearts

12 oz roasted and chopped red bell peppers

1/2 cup dry white wine

1/4 cup basil

1/2 cup whipping cream

3 tbsp drained capers

1 tsp grated lemon peel

3/4 cup feta cheese

2 tbsp lemon juice

2 oz toasted pine nuts

Directions :

Boil water in a pot and cook pasta in it.

Drain pasta and set aside.

Melt butter in a skillet over medium flame. Sauté garlic and cook for one minute.

Stir in shrimps and cook for about two minutes.

Mix artichokes, capers, bell pepper, and wine. Let it boil.

Lower the flame and let it simmer for two minutes with occasional stirring.

Add whipping cream, lemon juice, and lemon zest.

Let it boil for five minutes.

Transfer the cooked shrimps over pasta and mix well.

Spread cheese, basil, and nuts and serve.

Nutrition Info: Calories: 627 kcal Fat: 24 g Protein: 38 g Carbs: 58 g Fiber: 3 g

30 minutes Caprese chicken

Preparation time: 10 minutes
Cooking time: 20 minutes
Servings: 4

Ingredients:

Two boneless chicken breasts
Black pepper to taste
1 tbsp butter
1 tbsp extra virgin olive oil
6 oz Pesto
Eight chopped tomatoes
Six grated mozzarella cheese
Balsamic glaze as needed
Kosher salt to taste
Basil as required

Directions :

Mix salt, sliced chicken, and pepper in a bowl. Set aside for ten minutes.
Melt butter in a skillet over medium flame.
Cook chicken pieces in melted butter for five minutes from both sides.

Remove from the flame. Sprinkle pesto and place mozzarella cheese and tomatoes over chicken pieces. Bake in a preheated oven at 400 degrees for 12 minutes.

Garnish with balsamic glaze and serve.

Nutrition Info: Calories: 232 kcal Fat: 15 g Protein: 18 g Carbs: 5 g Fiber: 1 g

Greek turkey burgers with Tzatziki sauce

Preparation time: 36 minutes

Cooking time: 10 minutes

Servings: 4

Ingredients:

Turkey Burgers

1 lb ground turkey

1/3 cup chopped sun-dried tomatoes

½ cup chopped spinach leaves

1/4 cup chopped red onion

2 pressed garlic cloves

¼ cup feta cheese

One egg

1 tsp dried oregano

1 tbsp olive oil

1/2 tsp kosher salt

One sliced red onion

Four hamburger buns

1/2 tsp ground black pepper

A handful of Bibb lettuce leaves

Tzatziki Sauce

½ grated cucumber

Two minced garlic cloves

3/4 cup Greek yogurt

1 tbsp red wine vinegar

One pinch of kosher salt

1 tbsp chopped dill

One pinch of black pepper

Directions : Combine all the ingredients of Tzatziki sauce in a bowl and mix well.

Mix turkey, onion, sun-dried tomatoes, and feta cheese in a bowl.

In another bowl, mix olive oil, egg, garlic, salt, oregano, and pepper.

Pour egg mixture with turkey mixture. Mix well.

Make medium-sized patties out of turkey mixture. Set aside in the refrigerator for 24 hours.

Cook turkey patties on heated grill sprayed with oil for seven minutes from both sides on medium flame.

Spread Tzatziki sauce over buns and place lettuce, onions, and cooked patties and serve.

Nutrition Info: Calories: 389 kcal Fat: 13 g Protein: 40 g Carbs: 31 g Fiber: 4 g

Saucy Greek baked shrimp

Preparation time: 15 minutes
Cooking time: 20 minutes
Servings: 4

Ingredients:

2 tbsp chopped dill

1 lb shrimp

1/4 tsp kosher salt

1/2 tsp red pepper flakes

3 tbsp olive oil

Three minced garlic cloves

One chopped onion

15 oz crushed tomatoes

1/2 tsp ground cinnamon

1/2 tsp ground allspice

1/2 cup crumbled feta cheese

Directions :

Add salt, shrimps, and pepper in a bowl. Toss well and keep it aside.

Cook garlic and onions in heated olive oil over medium flame for five minutes.

Add spices and stir for half a minute.

Mix tomatoes and let it simmer for 20 minutes with occasional stirring.

Transfer the tomato mixture to the baking sheet and add shrimps to it. Spread cheese and bake in a preheated oven at 375 degrees for 20 minutes.

Drizzle dill and serve.

Nutrition Info: Calories: 190 kcal Fat: 5.2 g Protein: 25.9 g Carbs: 11.9 g Fiber: 5.2 g

www.ingramcontent.com/pod-product-compliance
Lightning Source LLC
Chambersburg PA
CBHW070730030426
42336CB00013B/1935